I0420202

DASH Diet for Beginners Cookbook

30 Healthy and Delicious Recipes (Includes 10 Bonus Recipes)

Copyright © 2015, Susan Rice

All rights Reserved. No part of this publication or the information in it may be quoted from or reproduced in any form by means such as printing, scanning, photocopying or otherwise without prior written permission of the copyright holder.

Disclaimer and Terms of Use:

Effort has been made to ensure that the information in this book is accurate and complete, however, the author and the publisher do not warrant the accuracy of the information, text and graphics contained within the book due to the rapidly changing nature of science, research, known and unknown facts and internet. The Author and the publisher do not hold any responsibility for errors, omissions or contrary interpretation of the subject matter herein. This book is presented solely for motivational and informational purposes only.

TABLE OF CONTENTS

Introduction

The DASH (Dietary Approaches to Stop Hypertension) diet focuses on long-term healthy eating habits. The diet doesn't make you starve or constantly crave. It works by controlling the size of the portions you eat, for each food group, making sure you get the optimal levels of potassium, calcium, magnesium, fiber and protein.

The DASH diet chooses certain food groups for specific reasons. Fruits and vegetables give you the magnesium and potassium your body needs. Low fat dairy products provide calcium. Each food you eat should have a purpose, and that's the principle of the DASH diet that is most important: eat well so you feel well.

Here are some additional details to remember when you're following the DASH principles:

a) Reduce the sodium in your diet. The diet recommends less than 2,300 mg of sodium per day. The National Heart, Lung and Blood Institute recommends lowering the sodium intake even further, to 1,500 mg, for people in the following groups: people with high blood pressure, people with diabetes or chronic kidney disease, African Americans, and people aged 51 and over.
b) Eat fruits, vegetables and low-fat dairy products
c) Eat high fiber foods
d) Focus on healthy fats that are good for your heart instead of saturated fats
e) Achieve and maintain a healthy body weight
f) Eat a lot of potassium and magnesium
g) Stay hydrated, particularly with water
h) Avoid smoking

How the DASH Diet Works

The DASH diet is really more than just a diet - it's a lifestyle.

There are numerous health benefits associated with the DASH diet. Weight loss is one of the most important benefits and a leading reason for why people adopt the DASH diet. It also brings down blood pressure, which is an important medical reason that people are advised to follow this eating plan. However, eating the foods prescribed by the DASH diet will have a lot of other health benefits that aren't as widely promoted. You'll get a lot more energy because your blood sugar will be stable and your metabolism will speed up. The fruits and veggies you fill up on will provide a lot of cancer-fighting and immune-boo sting antioxidants to your system. Many people report looking and feeling younger as well. If you have a history of diabetes in your family, the DASH diet can help reduce symptoms that may have already showed up.

Elevated blood pressure can cause a long list of health problems. You're at higher risk for having a heart attack or a stroke, and your heart is working a little too hard to keep up with the normal functions of your body. A major culprit is salt and sodium. That's the target of the DASH diet - to eliminate the excess sodium you have in your body and to replace it with nutrients that are far more beneficial. Foods rich in potassium and magnesium have been found to help your body reduce blood pressure naturally. Instead of popping pills, you can simply eat differently and live healthier.

What about Weight Loss?

Early versions of the DASH diet focused solely on blood pressure and didn't aim to help people lose weight. However, when patients following this eating plan began to lose weight naturally, people began to realize that it's a valuable weight loss tool as well. It's a great way to lose weight because it incorporates fresh, whole foods and reduces packaged, processed foods that are filled with empty calories. Not only will you lose weight, you'll also have a better chance of keeping it off. DASH goes beyond the calorie counting and helps you establish sound eating habits that are good for weight management.

Getting Started

Healthy, high fiber grains that are low in sugar is a good way to start on the DASH diet. These include whole grain cereals and breads, brown rice and even a little pasta. You should have four or five servings of fruits and vegetables every day. Recommended vegetables include lettuce, cabbage, celery, carrots, spinach, squash, broccoli, cucumbers, tomatoes, avocados, mushrooms and beans. Recommended fruits include blackberries, blueberries, strawberries, apples, pears, bananas, citrus fruits, melons and mango.

You can eat milk, yogurt and cheese too, just be sure to watch for added salt and sugar in these products. Nuts and legumes are also a big part of the DASH diet. Get your protein from lean sources of meat and eggs. In addition, the DASH diet encourages fish such as salmon, tilapia and mackerel.

It's essential to stay away from salt and trans fats when you're following the DASH diet. Use olive oil instead of butter and stick to healthy food preparations such as steaming and grilling. Keep sauces to a minimum and while snacking is encouraged, choose healthy snacks instead of processed foods that are high in calories and added sodium.

Changing your eating habits needs to be done gradually. Here are a few suggestions to help you make an easy transition to the DASH diet.

Keep a journal and track your eating habits. What do you eat for breakfast, lunch and dinner? How often do you eat in between meals and what are you snacking on? From your journal, you can see where you need to make changes. For example, add a cup or two of vegetables and fruits and reduce the servings of meat. Limit your sodium and sugar by reading the nutrition facts labels on food packages.

When shopping, choose "low-fat", "non-fat", "no sugar added", "no cholesterol" and other healthier versions of food. For grain servings, choose whole grains such as whole wheat bread or whole grain cereals.

If you love butter or margarine, decrease it by half and then switch to no-cholesterol and low-sodium versions. You can use spices as a substitute for salt. Experiment with different herbs if you're not sure how they taste. Some examples of spices are rosemary, basil, nutmeg, parsley, sage and thyme.

Recipes

Breakfast

Eggs with cheese

Egg whites are better than eggs, and this DASH diet recipe allows you to combine both.

Ingredients:

- 1 egg
- 2 egg whites
- 2 tablespoons fat-free milk
- 1 ounce grated cheddar cheese, reduced fat
- 1 green onion, chopped
- 1/4 cup tomato, chopped
- 2 slices whole wheat bread

Mix the egg and egg whites in a bowl and add the milk. Scramble the mixture in a non-stick frying pan until the eggs cook.

Meanwhile, toast the bread. Spoon the scrambled egg mixture onto the toasted bread and top with the cheese until it melts. Add the onion and the tomato.

Chicken breakfast burrito

Breakfast is the most important meal of the day and if you like to maximize your healthy food intake in the morning, this recipe is for you. To save time, you can cook the chicken the night before and keep it in the fridge.

Ingredients:

> 4 ounces cooked skinless chicken
>
> 1 whole wheat tortilla
>
> 1 cup fresh spinach
>
> 1 pear, sliced
>
> 2 tablespoons fat-free salad dressing

Slice the chicken into small bite-sized pieces and arrange them on the tortilla. Cover the meat with spinach and arrange the pear slices on top.

Drizzle with your choice of salad dressing - look for one that is fat-free; low calorie and low in sodium.

Wrap the tortilla around all the ingredients until it's a snug burrito.

Wheat bagel with apple

There's no need to give up your morning bagel when you're following the DASH plan. This recipe packs in some protein as well as whole grains and fruit.

Ingredients:

      1 whole wheat, whole grain bagel

      1 apple, sliced

      2 tablespoons natural peanut butter

Spread the peanut butter on each side of the bagel (make sure you use a brand that has no added salt) and layer the apple slices on top of the peanut butter.

Fruit and nut parfait

A perfect blend of crisp and crunch, you'll enjoy the creamy yogurt and the crunchy walnuts.

Ingredients:

  1 cup melon

  1 banana

  1 cup mixed berries

  1 /4 cup raisins

  1/2 cup walnuts

  2 cups fat free vanilla yogurt

Cut the melon into chunks that are about the same size as your berries and slice the banana. Mix in a large bowl with the raisins and the walnuts.

Top with the yogurt and blend to combine. Chill for about 30 minutes and serve in two separate bowls.

Mango smoothie

If you don't have a big appetite in the morning but you know you need to eat, try this smoothie.

Ingredients:

  1 cup frozen or fresh mango

  1 medium banana

  1/4 cup fat-free yogurt, plain

  1/2 cup fat-free milk

  1 cup kale

  1/4 cup whole oats

  1 cup ice

Place the milk, yogurt and oats in a blender and combine on low speed for 30 seconds.

Add the mango, banana, kale and ice and blend on high speed until smooth and combined. You can eliminate the ice if you don't want a smoothie that tastes too frozen.

This makes one smoothie and it's great for sticking with the DASH plan when you need to dash out the door in the mornings.

Grapefruit yogurt bowl

Get creative and put a new spin on your favorite fruit salad.

Ingredients:

  1/2 grapefruit

  1 cup strawberries, chopped

  1 teaspoon brown sugar

  1 cup fat-free vanilla yogurt

  1/4 cup walnuts

  1/4 cup blueberries

Scoop out the grapefruit segments from the rind and place in a bowl. Add the strawberries and blueberries and combine. Toss the fruit mixture with the brown sugar.

Place the yogurt in the hollow grapefruit shell. Spoon the fruit mixture onto the yogurt and sprinkle the top with walnuts.

Rice pilaf

This rice dish is inspired by South Asian pilau, which often include fruit and nuts, so it`s great for breakfast.

Ingredients:

> 2 1/4 cups vegetable stock
>
> 1 1/4 cups long grain brown rice
>
> 1/4 cup pistachios
>
> 1/4 cup dried apricots
>
> 3 tablespoons orange juice
>
> 1 1/2 tablespoons canola, coconut or sunflower oil
>
> 1/4 teaspoon saffron salt substitute to taste

Combine the rice, stock and saffron in a medium saucepan. Bring to a boil over high heat. Reduce the heat to low and cover, simmering until the rice has become tender and absorbed all the liquid. Transfer to a large bowl.

Combine the orange juice, oil and salt substitute in a small bowl. Pour this mixture over the rice.

Chop the apricots.

Heat a small skillet to medium and add the fruit and nuts, stirring continuously until the pistachios brown slightly and develop an oily appearance.

Toss the fruit and nuts with the flavored rice to mix.

Serve right away.

Homemade granola

This homemade granola recipe is nutritionally dense and concentrates on healthy fats and natural, relatively unrefined sources of sugar.

Ingredients:

3 cups old-fashioned rolled oats

1 cup sliced almonds

1 cup raisins or dried cranberries

4 tablespoons flax seed

1/4 cup raw sugar

1/4 cup honey

1/4 cup sunflower or canola oil

1/2 teaspoon vanilla extract

1/2 teaspoon ground sugar

1/2 teaspoon allspice

1/2 teaspoon ground ginger

Combine the oats, almonds, flax, spices and sugar in a large bowl, mixing thoroughly.

In a separate bowl combine the honey, oil and vanilla extract. Pour the wet ingredient mixture into the dry ingredients, mixing with a spatula as you pour. Stir until the dry mixture is wet throughout.

Lightly grease one to two cookie sheets with sunflower oil or another monounsaturated fat. Pour the wet granola into the pans, patting it into place if necessary.

Bake in a 250 degree Fahrenheit oven for 90 minutes or until dry and lightly browned, stirring every 15 minutes. Break up chunks of granola as you stir to create the appropriate consistency.

Allow the mixture to cool, then combine with the dried fruit and store in an air-tight container.

Breakfast sandwich

If you love eggs for breakfast, this recipe will help you enjoy them without the heart risk associated with large amounts of egg yolk. Flavorful mustard and tomatoes keep the open-faced sandwich interesting, so you won't miss the fat.

Ingredients:

> 2 egg whites
>
> 1/2 cup fresh spinach leaves
>
> 1 slice whole grain bread
>
> 1 small tomato
>
> 1 1/2 teaspoons olive oil
>
> 1 teaspoon prepared brown mustard
>
> 1/2 ounce slice reduced-fat cheddar cheese
>
> Black pepper and paprika to taste

In a small pan, heat the olive oil to medium-high. Beat the egg whites and add to the hot oil, scrambling them until completely solid. Add the spinach and heat until wilted.

Spread the mustard onto the bread and place it on an oven-safe plate or baking sheet. Arrange tomato slices on top of the mustard, then top with the egg mixture and thinly-sliced cheddar cheese. Sprinkle with black pepper and sharp paprika to taste.

Bake in an oven or toaster oven at 400 degrees Fahrenheit until the bread is crisp and the cheese is melted and slightly browned.

Almond-banana toast

Putting the finished product under the broiler caramelizes the natural sugars in the banana, producing a delicious, gooey result that you'll also enjoy as a snack.

Ingredients:

> 2 slices whole grain bread
>
> 2 tablespoons smooth almond butter
>
> 1 small banana
>
> ground cinnamon and nutmeg to taste

Toast the bread and arrange it on an oven-safe plate or a small baking sheet. Spread each slice with 1 tablespoon of almond butter.

Slice the banana into rounds of medium thickness and arrange them on top of the almond butter.

Sprinkle the surface with cinnamon and nutmeg, then place under the broiler for 2 to 3 minutes, or until the almond butter melts slightly and the bananas begin to brown.

Allow to cool and eat with your fingers, or dig in right away with a fork.

Lunch

Brown rice and beans

If you like Caribbean food, this is a must for you, and even if you don't, please give it a try.

Ingredients:

   1 cup dark brown rice

   2 cups water

   1 teaspoon salt

   3 tablespoons fresh orange juice

   1 tablespoon olive oil

   1/4 cup pine nuts

   1 cup black beans, no salt added

   3 stems fresh cilantro

Combine rice, water, salt, olive oil in a saucepan and simmer for about 45 minutes, until rice cooks.

Remove from heat and add pine nuts and orange juice. Stir in the black beans until combined. Top with fresh cilantro.

This recipe serves 6.

Tantalizing tuna melt

This is easy-to-make lunch recipe. Plus, you can pack it for take away!

Ingredients:

4 whole wheat flour tortillas

2 cans of chunk light tuna in water, drained

8 tomato slices

1/4 cup red onion, chopped

1/4 cup celery, chopped

2 tablespoons lemon juice

2 tablespoons extra virgin olive oil

2 slices low-fat mozzarella cheese

Ground black pepper

Empty the tuna out of the cans into a small bowl. Use a fork to mix it with the olive oil and lemon juice.

Add the celery and the onion. Sprinkle pepper into the mixture.

Preheat your oven to 325 degrees. Lay the tortillas on a cookie sheet and spoon the tuna mixture onto each one, dividing it evenly. Top each with two thick tomato slices and then cover with cheese.

Bake for about 10 minutes, until the cheese is melted. Remove from oven and let cool for 2 minutes. Roll the tortilla into a wrap and enjoy.

This recipe makes four tuna melts.

Pear and walnut salad

Not your usual salad but the combination of pear and walnut gives so much pleasure and a wonderful sweet-salty taste.

Ingredients:

6 cups of mixed lettuces and greens

3 pears, thinly sliced

1/4 cup toasted walnuts, chopped

1 fennel bulb, thinly sliced

2 tablespoons grated pecorino cheese

3 tablespoons extra virgin olive oil

3 tablespoons balsamic vinegar

Ground black pepper

Wash the lettuces and place in a large bowl. Spread the fennel and the pear over the lettuces and top with the cheese, oil, vinegar and pepper. Finish with the chopped walnuts.

This recipe serves 4 people.

Pasta Primavera

Pasta Primavera means pasta with fresh vegetables, so you always use the fresh vegetables of the season.

Ingredients:

12 ounces whole wheat pasta

1 garlic clove, chopped

1 red bell pepper, chopped

1 green bell pepper, chopped

1 yellow bell pepper, chopped

1 cucumber, chopped

1 red onion, chopped

1 can diced tomatoes, no salt added

2 tablespoons extra virgin olive oil

1 tablespoon lemon juice

1/2 teaspoon basil

1/2 teaspoon oregano

1/2 teaspoon rosemary

1/2 teaspoon parsley

Cook the pasta and drain. Rinse with cool water and shake in a strainer until excess water is removed. Pour into a large bowl. Add olive oil and lemon juice, toss pasta to coat.

Add the chopped vegetables and combine. Sprinkle with herbs and pour the can of tomatoes on the top, juices included.

Allow the salad to chill in the refrigerator for at least one hour. Serve alone or on top of large lettuce leaves.

This recipe provides four generous servings.

Chicken chili

Not your usual chili, I admit. (I mean, chicken in a chili?!) But thanks to the slow cooking process and the different veggies and spices, you won't notice a difference.

Ingredients:

> 10 ounces skinless chicken, cooked
>
> 28 ounces canned crushed tomatoes, no salt added
>
> 2 cups black beans, no salt added
>
> 1 red onion, diced
>
> 2 stalks of celery, diced
>
> 1 red bell pepper, diced
>
> 2 jalapeno peppers, diced
>
> 2 cloves of garlic, minced
>
> 2 tablespoons red pepper flakes
>
> 1 tablespoon black pepper
>
> 1 tablespoon oregano
>
> 1 tablespoon olive oil
>
> 1/4 cup water

In a large soup pot, cook the celery, onion, peppers and garlic in the olive oil for 5 minutes.

Add all remaining ingredients and cook, covered for 2 hours. Stir occasionally while it simmers.

This recipe makes 8 servings.

Citrus shrimp salad

Here is a simple gourmet salad recipe with an orange twist.

Ingredients:

> 1/2 pound cooked small salad shrimp, peeled and rinsed
>
> 1/4 cup freshly squeezed orange juice
>
> 1 tablespoon balsamic vinegar
>
> 6 cups spinach and lettuce mix
>
> 1 cucumber, chopped
>
> 2 oranges, peeled and chopped

Combine the shrimp with the orange juice, vinegar and cucumber and toss. Chill the mixture in the refrigerator for at least 30 minutes.

Place the mixture on top of the lettuce and spinach and sprinkle with orange segments.

This recipe provides 4 salad servings.

Turkey salad sandwich

A healthy DASH version of one of the most popular sandwich choices in the world.

Ingredients:

2 slices whole grain bread

1/2 cup shredded turkey

1 tablespoon fat free mayonnaise

1/4 cup chopped celery

1/4 cup chopped apple

1 large lettuce leaf

2 tomato slices

Ground black pepper

Mix the shredded turkey in a bowl with mayonnaise, celery, apple and ground pepper.

Lay the lettuce leaf on top of one bread piece. Scoop the turkey out of the bowl and onto the lettuce leaf. Top with the tomato slices and place the other piece of bread on top.

This recipe creates one turkey sandwich.

Carrot curry

This smooth curry contains plenty of exciting spices, along with protein-rich low fat yogurt and bright, tangy cilantro. For a spicier version, substitute cayenne or Thai peppers for the jalapeno.

Ingredients:

5 cups low-sodium vegetable stock

1 pound carrots

1 large yellow onion

1 jalapeno pepper

1/4 cup cilantro leaves

1/4 cup low fat unsweetened yogurt

2 tablespoons lime or lemon juice

1 tablespoon sunflower oil

1 tablespoon fresh ginger

2 cloves garlic

2 teaspoons Madras curry powder

1 teaspoon black mustard seeds salt substitute to taste

Heat the olive oil in a large saucepan to medium.

Mince the garlic and ginger and chop the onion finely.

Add the mustard seed to the oil and allow it to pop, then add the ginger, garlic and onion. Cook for about 5 minutes, stirring continuously, or until the onions become translucent but not brown.

Remove the stem, seeds and ribs of the jalapeno and chop it finely, then add to the pan along with the curry powder.

Chop the carrots roughly and sauté with the other ingredients for about 3 minutes, or until the seasonings begin to toast. Pour in about half of the stock and bring the whole pot to a boil over high heat. Reduce to medium-low and simmer for about 5 minutes, or until the carrots become tender.

Remove the soup from the pot and place it in a blender or food processor. Process until the liquid is smooth, in batches if necessary, and return to the pan. Stir in the remaining stock and reheat.

Add yogurt, cilantro and lime juice, as well as salt substitute to taste. Garnish with additional cilantro and limes before serving.

Edamame salad

Fresh, steamed soybeans are known as Edamame in Japan, and are eaten as an appetizer or part of other dishes. When served cold, these beans also make a great salad ingredient.

Ingredients:

>   1/2 pound fresh Edamame
>
>   1 pint cherry or grape tomatoes
>
>   1/4 cup red wine vinegar
>
>   1 1/2 tablespoons extra virgin olive oil
>
>   1 scallion
>
>   1 small bunch fresh dill weed
>
>   1 small bunch fresh mint
>
>   1/4 teaspoon black pepper

Place the soybeans in a steamer over about an inch of water. Cover and steam for approximately 5 minutes, or until the pods are bright green and the beans are crisp-tender. Rinse with cold water and remove from the pods.

Set the beans aside in a medium bowl and refrigerate.

Chop the mint and dill finely. Slice the green onion. Cut large cherry tomatoes into halves, leaving small ones whole.

Combine tomatoes, green onion, mint and dill in a medium bowl.

Mix oil, vinegar and black pepper in a small bowl and pour over the salad.

Serve chilled.

DASH pasta sauce

The DASH diet works best when you reduce the amount of meat in your diet, but many people don't know where to start. This vegetable-based pasta sauce proves that you don't need to have sausage or beef to make a meal special. Serve it with your favorite whole grain pasta.

Ingredients:

> 8 ounces canned low-sodium tomato sauce
>
> 6 ounces canned low-sodium tomato paste
>
> 2 medium zucchini
>
> 2 medium fresh tomatoes
>
> 2 small onions
>
> 3 cloves garlic
>
> 2 tablespoons olive oil
>
> 1 tablespoon dried oregano
>
> 1 tablespoon dried basil
>
> 1 teaspoon dried rosemary
>
> 1 cup water

Heat the olive oil in a medium-sized skillet.

Mince the garlic and onions. Chop the zucchini and tomatoes coarsely.

Add all vegetables to the pan and sauté for about 5 minutes over medium-high heat, or until the onions become slightly translucent.

Mix the tomato paste and water in a medium bowl until smooth. Add to the pan, along with the tomato sauce and herbs. Cover and reduce the heat to low. Simmer for 45 minutes or until the sauce reaches the desired consistency.

Season with salt substitute if desired.

Dinner

Salmon salad

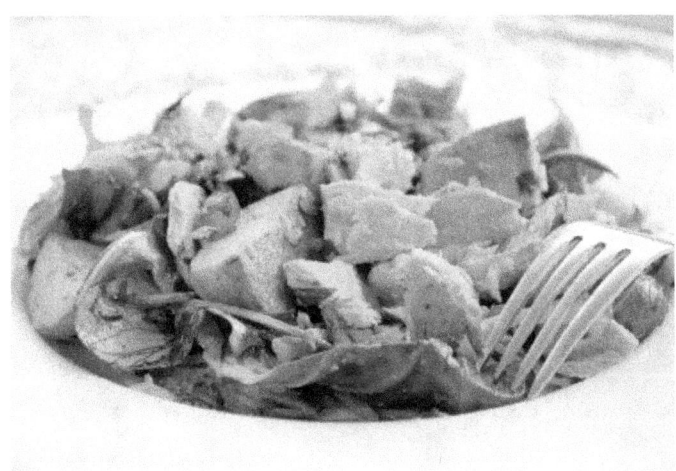

A quick and easy dinner recipe which has amazing anti-inflammatory effects, especially if you use wild salmon.

Ingredients:

4 salmon filets, 6 ounces each

2 tablespoons lemon juice

1 garlic clove, minced

8 lemon slices

2 tablespoons fresh Italian parsley

ground black pepper

6 cups mixed lettuce greens

2 tomatoes, chopped

1/4 cup toasted almonds, salt-free

1/4 cup extra virgin olive oil

Preheat the oven to 350 degrees. Cover the salmon with lemon juice, garlic and lemon slices. Sprinkle with parsley and pepper and cook for 15 minutes.

Mix the salad with lettuce, tomatoes, almonds and olive oil. Place the salmon on top.

This recipe serves 4.

Chicken kebab

This Middle East inspired recipe is perfect for the BBQ in summer.

Ingredients:

> 12 ounces cooked chicken, cut into pieces
>
> 2 red bell peppers, chopped
>
> 1 red onion, chopped
>
> 2 cups cherry or grape tomatoes
>
> 1 cup button mushrooms
>
> 1 cup pineapple chunks
>
> 2 tablespoons olive oil
>
> Ground black pepper

Heat a grill or a grill pan and place the meat, vegetables and pineapple chunks on skewers in any pattern that appeals to you.

Brush each kebab with olive oil and sprinkle with pepper. Heat the kebabs on the grill, turning to ensure all sides are cooked. Remove from the grill and serve with a side of salad or a bowl of fruit.

This recipe serves 4 people (2 kebabs each).

Turkey burgers

Okay, it's actually not a burger per se but once you have tasted it, you will never ever again look for the big yellow M signs by the road.

Ingredients:

> 1 pound ground turkey breast
>
> 1/3 cup whole grain oats
>
> 4 slices whole grain wheat bread
>
> 4 slices low fat cheddar cheese
>
> 1 cup raw spinach leaves
>
> 1 tomato, sliced
>
> 1/4 red onion, sliced into rings
>
> Ground black pepper
>
> 1/4 cup chopped yellow onion
>
> 1/4 cup chopped red pepper
>
> 2 tablespoons fat free mayonnaise

Put the red pepper and yellow onion in a food processor and pulse until very fine. Combine with the turkey breast and the whole oats.

Heat a grill or a grill pan. While the grill heats up, form the turkey mixture into 4 patties of equal size. Grill on each side, until cooked and allow the cheese to melt before you remove from grill.

While they are cooking, toast the bread. Spread a light layer of mayonnaise on the bread and place one turkey patty on each slice. Top with spinach, tomato and red onion. Sprinkle with black pepper.

This makes four turkey burgers.

BBQ chops

Barbecued pork may sound unhealthy and decadent, but you can substitute other meats to make your favorite pork recipes compatible with the DASH diet. This recipe uses "chops" of boneless chicken thighs, since the dark meat provides similar flavor intensity to that of lean pork. Add a fresh salad and this dish is ready to make a complete meal!

Ingredients:

> 1 1/2 pounds boneless chicken thighs
>
> 10 ounces low sodium condensed tomato soup
>
> 3 tablespoons red wine vinegar
>
> 2 tablespoons low sodium
>
> Worcestershire sauce
>
> 1 small onion
>
> 3/4 cup water
>
> 1 teaspoon sharp paprika
>
> 1 teaspoon chili powder
>
> 1/4 teaspoon cinnamon
>
> 1/4 teaspoon black pepper
>
> 1/8 teaspoon cloves

Trim all fat from the chicken, cube, and set aside.

Combine all other ingredients in a large bowl, then transfer to a large skillet with high sides.

Heat to medium and add the chicken cubes, simmering for 30 minutes or until cooked thoroughly.

Serve with bread or 2/3 cup of brown rice.

Blackened beef

Thinly sliced lean top round beef seared with strong spices makes for an exciting and flavorful main dish, especially when you pair it with stewed potatoes, onions and carrots

Ingredients:

1 pound lean top round of beef

6 medium red potatoes

4 large onions

3 large carrots

2 cups low-sodium beef broth

2 cups water

2 cloves garlic

1 bunch kale

2 tablespoons sharp paprika

1 tablespoon dried oregano

1 teaspoon chili powder

1 teaspoon powdered garlic

1/2 teaspoon black pepper

1/4 teaspoon red pepper

1/4 teaspoon mustard powder

Place the beef in the freezer until partially frozen.

Cut the potatoes into quarters, mince the garlic cloves, slice the carrots into rounds and remove the stems from the kale.

Chop the onions very finely to yield about 4 cups.

Combine paprika, oregano, garlic powder, chili powder, red and black peppers and dry mustard in a small bowl with a lid. Set aside.

Remove beef from freezer and slice it across the grain in strips about 1/8 inch thick. Sprinkle with the seasoning mix, covering all available surfaces.

Lightly grease a large heavy skillet or stockpot then preheat over high. Add the meat strips and sear, stirring continuously, for about 5 minutes.

Add the broth and water to the pan to deglaze, then add potatoes and garlic to the skillet. Allow the blackened spices to float to the top.

Cover and lower heat to medium, cooking for about 20 minutes or until potatoes are tender.

Add the carrots and place the kale on top of the dish. Cover and cook for an additional 10 minutes.

This dish can be served right from the skillet or pot.

Greek pizza

Many DASH dieters find that they miss conventional pizza after they start their new healthier way of eating. Once you learn to make these pizzas at home, you won't miss delivery.

Ingredients:

10 ounces fresh or frozen spinach

3 1/4 cups low sodium marinara sauce

1 1/4 cups reduced-fat ricotta cheese

1 1/4 cups fresh mint

1 cup fresh fennel

1 whole grain 14 inch pizza crust or equivalent dough

3/4 cup feta cheese crumbles

4 plum tomatoes

1 teaspoon strongly-flavored olive oil

1 teaspoon cornmeal

salt substitute and black pepper to taste

Heat a pizza stone or cookie sheet in the oven at 500 degrees Fahrenheit. Sprinkle a pizza peel with cornmeal to prevent sticking. If you are using a pizza crust, follow package instructions to prepare it for topping.

Chop the mint, tomatoes, fennel and spinach.

Heat the olive oil in a large skillet to medium-high.

Add the chopped fennel and sauté for five minutes, or until slightly translucent. Reduce the heat to medium-low.

Drain all water from the spinach and add it to the fennel. Season with black pepper and salt substitute according to your preferences.

Place the raw dough on the pizza peel and transfer it to the baking stone or sheet.

Cook for 5 minutes at 500 degrees and remove from oven.

Spread the sauce over the pizza crust, then top with the spinach and fennel mixture. Spoon the ricotta in small quantities over the vegetable mixture, but do not try to spread it.

Add feta crumbles and bake for another 15 minutes, or until the crust is cooked completely and the edges are lightly browned.

Combine the mint and tomatoes in a separate bowl, then sprinkle them over the surface of the pizza before cutting.

Lentil chili

This tasty vegetarian alternative to conventional chili is hearty and flavorful, with bulgur wheat and lentils replacing the usual fatty beef and chili beans.

Ingredients:

> 3 cups low-sodium vegetable broth
>
> 2 cups or one can chopped tomatoes
>
> 1 cup bulgur wheat
>
> 1 cup dried lentils
>
> 1 medium white onion
>
> 4 cloves garlic
>
> 2 tablespoons canola oil
>
> 2 1/2 tablespoons chili powder
>
> 1 tablespoon cumin powder
>
> 1/2 teaspoon cinnamon
>
> Salt substitute and pepper to taste

Heat the oil to medium-high in a large pot.

Mince the onion and garlic, then add them to the pot and cook for 5 minutes, stirring continuously. When the alliums have become slightly translucent, add the wheat and lentils, followed by the broth.

Stir to combine, then add the tomatoes and spices.

Bring to a boil over high heat, then reduce to low and cover. Simmer for 30 minutes or until the lentils just begin to fall apart.

Add salt substitute and pepper to taste and serve hot.

Grilled chicken

This basic chicken dish is easy to make on any outdoor grill. You won't miss the extra fat!

Ingredients:

       4 bone-in chicken breasts with skin

       2 cloves garlic

       salt-free herb seasoning mix

Heat a gas or charcoal grill to medium heat.

Fold non-stick aluminum foil into a boat shape for each chicken breast.

Cut the garlic cloves in half and rub the cut surfaces over the skin of the chicken breasts. Sprinkle with seasoning mix to taste and place the chicken breasts in the boats, skin side down.

Grill for 45 minutes or until the center reaches 160 degrees Fahrenheit, turning the chicken once every 10 to 15 minutes.

Asian cod

This spicy Asian fish recipe provides plenty of healthy polyunsaturated omega-3 fatty acids, along with the rich flavors of miso and chili paste. If cod is unavailable, use any firm, flaky white fish that can be cut into thick steaks.

Ingredients:

1 pound cod

3 tablespoons low-salt sweet white miso

1 tablespoon garlic-chili paste

2 tablespoons apple juice

2 tablespoons unprocessed cane sugar, such as turbinado

Mix together all raw ingredients except for the fish.

Take a piece of plastic wrap and spread it over the counter or a cutting board, then apply a layer of miso marinade a little larger than the total surface area of the fish.

Place a piece of cheesecloth on top of the marinade layer. Wrap the cheesecloth around the fish, then apply marinade to the top side. Wrap the plastic around the fish and its wrapping, then place the plastic bundle into a freezer bag.

Place in the refrigerator for two hours to overnight.

Remove the fish from the refrigerator and peel away the plastic and cheesecloth layers.

Heat a large nonstick frying pan over medium heat and place the fish in it. Cook on both sides until the fish is opaque and flaky throughout.

Serve with low-sodium miso soup, rice and Japanese pickles.

Discard any unused marinade for safety reasons.

Chinese beef

This dish uses thinly-sliced lean beef, heart-friendly oils and fresh ginger to recreate a classic Chinese restaurant favorite.

Ingredients:

3/4 pound thinly-sliced flank or sirloin steak

1 medium onion

1 pound mushrooms

1 pound broccoli

2 tablespoons peanut oil

1 tablespoon rice vinegar

1 tablespoon fresh ginger

3 cloves fresh garlic

red pepper flakes to taste

salt substitute to taste

In a deep skillet or wok, heat 1 tablespoon of peanut oil on high.

Mince the ginger and onion and add to the hot pan, frying for about a minute.

Season with salt substitute to taste.

Crush the garlic, slice the mushrooms and chop the broccoli. Add 1 teaspoon of garlic and the mushrooms to the pan.

Cook for about 2 minutes, stirring throughout, or until the mushrooms soften and the onions become translucent.

Add the broccoli and cook for about 3 minutes or until it is bright green and still slightly crisp.

Remove the vegetables to a bowl.

Add the remaining tablespoon of peanut oil to the pan and allow it to heat.

Add the beef strips and the remaining garlic, cooking for about 2 minutes. Sprinkle in the vinegar and red pepper flakes, followed by the vegetables. Stir to combine and remove from the heat immediately.

Serve over short grain brown rice.

Conclusion

If you're worried that your health could be at risk, it's time to take steps.

That means moving to the DASH diet and avoiding unhealthy foods in favor of rich, flavorful options that are low in fat and high in vitamins. While it's true that the adjustment period may take a little longer than you expect, all these recipes will help you make the transition.

You won't miss the fat or extra sugar! Just focus on the healthy foods that you can eat and work to make fruits and vegetables a regular part of your routine. Your heart and your waistline will thank you.

Bon appétit!

Bonus Recipes

TABLE OF CONTENTS

Grilled pineapple

Ingredients:

  1 firm and ripe pineapple

  1 tablespoon dark rum

  1 tablespoon fresh lime juice

  2 tablespoons dark honey

  1 tablespoon olive oil

  1 tablespoon grated lime zest

  1/4 teaspoon ground cloves

  1 teaspoon ground cinnamon

Prepare the grill for high heat.

To make the marinade, combine the olive oil, cinnamon, cloves, limejuice and honey in a large bowl.

Cut the crown of leaves and the base of the pineapple. While keeping the pineapple standing upright, use a large sharp knife to pare off the skin, cutting downward just below the surface in vertical strips. Cut the pineapple, into half lengthwise then place each pineapple half cut side down and cut into four long wedges; remove the core.

Place the pineapple in the bowl with the marinade and stir to coat the pineapple.

Place on the grill and cook for around four minutes, as you baste with the remaining marinade. Turn the fruit and move it to a cooler part of the grill then reduce the heat. Baste again with the marinade and grill until the pineapple is tender and golden brown. This should take around three minutes.

Remove the pineapple from the grill, place on a platter and brush with the rum then sprinkle with the zest. You can serve either warm or hot.

Fruit kebabs with lemon dip

Ingredients:

4 to 6 strawberries

4 to 6 pineapple chunks

4 to 6 grapes

1/2 banana cut into chunks

1 kiwi, peeled and diced

1 teaspoon lime zest

1 teaspoon fresh lime juice

4 ounces low fat, sugar free lemon yogurt

Whisk together the yogurt, lime zest and lime juice. Cover and refrigerate until when needed.

Thread one of each fruit on the skewer. Serve with the lemon lime dip.

Banana oatmeal pancakes with maple syrup

Ingredients:

1 banana, mashed

1/2 cup rolled oats

1/2 cup maple syrup

1 cup water

3 whole cloves

1/2 cinnamon stick

2 tablespoons canola oil

2 tablespoons light brown sugar

1/2 cup all-purpose flour

1/2 cup whole wheat flour

1/3 teaspoons baking soda

1/3 teaspoon ground cinnamon

1 1/2 teaspoons baking powder

1/2 cup fat-free plain yogurt

1/2 cup low-fat milk

1 egg, lightly beaten

1/2 teaspoon salt

Combine the maple syrup, cloves and cinnamon stick in a saucepan.

Place the pan over medium heat and bring to a boil. Remove from the heat and allow it to steep for 15 minutes. Remove the cloves and cinnamon stick with a spoon and set the syrup aside then keep warm.

Combine oats and water in a microwave-safe bowl and microwave on high until the oats are tender and creamy. Stir in canola oil and brown sugar and put aside to cool.

Combine the flours, baking soda, baking powder, ground cinnamon and salt. Whisk to ensure it is well blended.

Add milk, banana and yogurt to the oats and stir in until well blended. Beat in the egg, add the flour mixture to the oat mixture, and stir until moistened.

Place a frying pan over medium heat and once hot, spoon 1/3 cup batter into the pan. Cook until the top surface is covered with bubbles and the edges lightly browned. Turn and cook until the bottom is well brown. Repeat with the remaining batter.

Place the pancakes on warmed plates, drizzle with warm syrup, and serve.

Fruit crunch

Ingredients:

4 cups assorted fresh fruit like grapefruit, orange, chopped pear, seedless grapes, cubed fresh pineapple and sliced kiwi fruit

2 tablespoons honey

1/2 cup low fat granola

2 cans (6 ounces each) low fat yogurt

1/4 cup coconut toasted

Divide the fruit into 6 parfait glasses or bowls

Top the fruit with yoghurt and drizzle with honey.

Sprinkle with coconut and granola.

Yogurt with fresh strawberries and honey

Ingredients:

   3 cups plain low-fat yogurt

   4 tablespoons toasted sliced almonds

   4 teaspoons honey

   1 pint fresh strawberries

Clean and slice the strawberries into quarters then set aside

Place 3/4 cup of the yogurt into four serving dishes.

Divide the strawberries evenly among the dishes.

Top each with a teaspoon of honey then a teaspoon of toasted almonds.

Serve immediately.

Milk chocolate pudding

Ingredients:

   2 tablespoons cocoa powder

   3 tablespoons cornstarch

   1/8 teaspoon salt

   2 tablespoons sugar

   2 cups non-fat milk

   1/2 teaspoon vanilla

   1/3 cup chocolate chips

Mix the cornstarch, sugar, cocoa powder and sugar in a saucepan until well mixed then add in milk and whisk.

Heat over medium heat as you continue stirring frequently until it thickens.

Remove from heat and stir in vanilla and the chocolate chips until melted and smooth.

Pour into a large dish and chill. Place plastic wrap over the surface to prevent a skin from forming on top.

Mixed berry pie

Ingredients:

3/4 cup raspberries

12 strawberries, sliced

1/2 cup fat free, sugar free instant vanilla pudding made using low-fat or fat-free milk

6 tablespoons light whipped topping

6 single serve graham cracker pie crusts

6 mint leaves for garnishing

Mix the raspberries and strawberries in a small bowl.

Spoon 4 teaspoons of the pudding into every pie crust. Add the two tablespoons of the raspberry-strawberry mixture into each pie. Top with one tablespoon of whipped topping and garnish with mint leaves.

Serve immediately.

Grapes and walnuts with sour cream

Ingredients:

1 1/2 cups red seedless grapes

3 tablespoons chopped walnuts

1/2 cup fat-free sour cream

2 tablespoons powdered sugar

1/2 teaspoon lemon juice

1/2 teaspoon lemon zest

1/8 teaspoon vanilla extract

Combine sour cream, lemon zest, powdered sugar, vanilla and lemon juice. Whisk, then cover and chill for several hours.

Divide the grapes among 6 dessert bowls then add two tablespoons of the lemon topping on every dish and sprinkle each bowl with 1/2 tablespoon of chopped walnuts.

Serve immediately.

Chocolate pie

Ingredients:

4 oz. white chocolate, finely chopped

1/4 cup sugar

1/2 lb cream cheese

1/2 cup heavy cream, chilled

1/3 cup sour cream

1 banana, sliced

1 readymade graham cracker crust around 9 inches

1 teaspoon vanilla extract

Warm the chocolate in a bowl over a pot of simmering water. When partially melted, remove from the heat and stir to melt completely.

Beat the sugar, vanilla and cream cheese until smooth. Beat in the sour cream and chocolate.

Whip the heavy cream until firm then gently fold into the chocolate filling.

Put the banana slices on the crust and top with the filling then chill for two hours. You can sprinkle with dark chocolate before serving.

Berry banana ice cream

Ingredients:

1 cup frozen berries

3 bananas cut into one inch pieces and frozen

1 1/2 teaspoons vanilla extract

1/2 cup non-fat milk

Put the frozen bananas in a food processor. Add milk and vanilla and process for one minute.

Once a smooth consistency has been achieved, add the berries and pulse until they are in pieces and incorporated into the banana mixture.

Serve immediately.

www.ingramcontent.com/pod-product-compliance
Lightning Source LLC
Chambersburg PA
CBHW081118280526
45787CB00007B/2888